AF207242

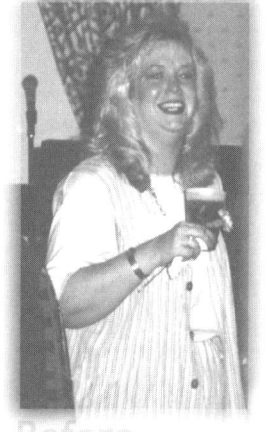

Before

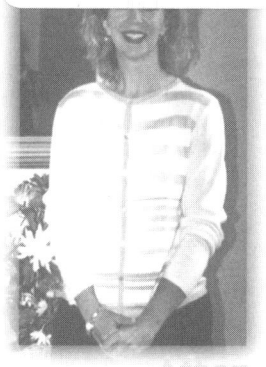

After

Abby Meloy

Pastor's Wife
Lake City, Florida

It has been five years since I began the First Place program, and today I am one truly thankful woman. I had been at the 200-pound mark (and over) for seven years. Now my weight stays around 135 pounds and I wear size 8 clothes.

In the beginning, I did not want to try First Place. I had no desire to weigh my food or take the time to learn the measurements, but since some women at my church wanted the program—and since I was a size 18/20—I thought I'd give it a shot. After my first three-month session, I was 27 pounds lighter. It took me nine months and three sessions to lose 74 pounds.

My favorite Scripture used in the program is Deuteronomy 30:11: "Now what I am commanding you today is not too difficult for you or beyond your reach."

I am now truly a new creature. My new lifestyle has inspired my husband to lose 20 pounds and my 13-year-old daughter to lose 35 pounds that she needed to lose. As a result, we are able to carry out the work of our ministry with much less fatigue. I now teach others in my church the First Place program and will be forever grateful that the Lord brought it into my life.

———

Rena Schaeffer

Atlanta, Texas

"My weight began to increase as my lifestyle changed after the birth of my two children. Before I knew it, my weight had skyrocketed to 219 pounds. I went to a First Place meeting and my life has never been the same. I lost 40 pounds in one three-month session. It can be done!"

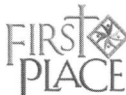
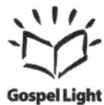

FIRST TASTE

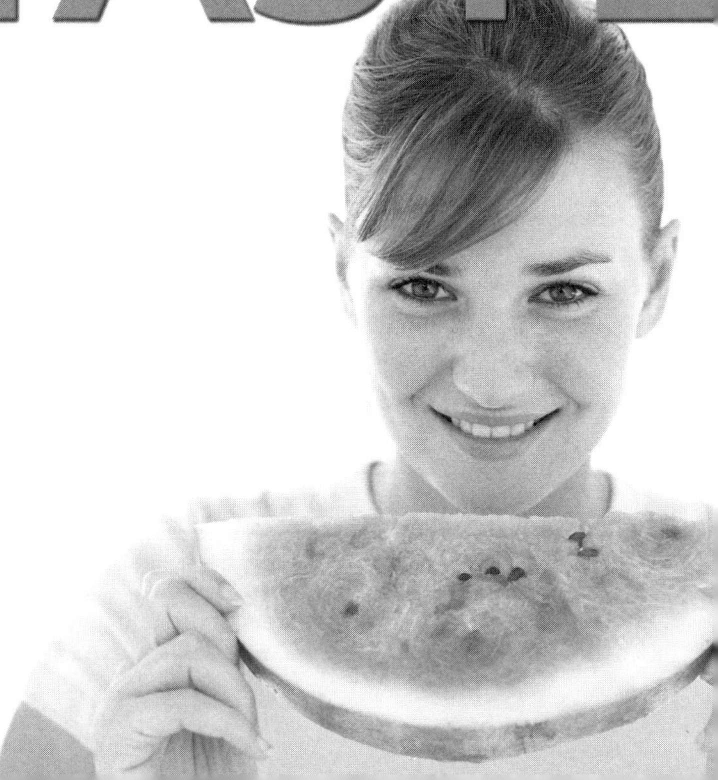

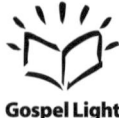

Gospel Light

Gospel Light is a Christian publisher dedicated to serving the local church. We believe God's vision for Gospel Light is to provide church leaders with biblical, user-friendly materials that will help them evangelize, disciple and minister to children, youth and families.

It is our prayer that this Gospel Light resource will help you discover biblical truth for your own life and help you minister to others. May God richly bless you.

For a free catalog of resources from Gospel Light, please contact your Christian supplier or contact us at 1-800-4-GOSPEL or www.gospellight.com.

PUBLISHING STAFF
William T. Greig, Publisher • **Dr. Elmer L. Towns,** Senior Consulting Publisher • **Bayard Taylor, M.Div.,** Senior Editor, Biblical and Theological Issues

ISBN 0-8307-3809-6
© 2005 First Place
All rights reserved.
Printed in the U.S.A.

Scripture quotations are taken from the *Holy Bible, New International Version®.* Copyright © 1973, 1978, 1984 by International Bible Society. Used by permission of Zondervan Publishing House. All rights reserved.

CAUTION

The information contained in this book is intended to be solely informational and educational. It is assumed that the First Place participant will consult a medical or health professional before beginning this or any other weight-loss or physical fitness program.

CONTENTS

WELCOME TO FIRST PLACE

The First Place program is the result of a godly desire placed in the hearts of a group of Christians to establish a Christ-centered weight-control program.

With that desire in mind, they began to develop a program that would meet the needs of Christians who needed to get their weight under control. It was an immense assignment, but knowing God had called them to the task, they placed all of their hopes and aspirations in Him and began the project. They prayed, studied, prayed, read, prayed, wrote—and First Place began to take shape!

They knew that the program needed to include Bible study, small-group support, accountability, a proven commonsense nutrition plan, exercise, record keeping and many other elements to be effective. They knew putting Christ first in their lives would be the success of the program. Their aim was for growth in all areas of a person's life: spiritual, mental, emotional and physical.

Matthew 6:33, "Seek first his kingdom and his righteousness, and all these things will be given to you as well," was chosen as the theme verse for the program. Hence, the name First Place.

The original First Place groups met in the spring of 1981 at First Baptist Church of Houston, Texas. What began as a Christ-centered weight-loss program has evolved into a nationally recognized total health program. Today the First Place program is used in every state and in many foreign countries. Thousands of lives have been changed radically through the power of Christ.

We praise God for the leadership He provided as all of the steps of First Place were planned and penned. Our greatest desire continues to be, that God will receive all the glory, honor and praise and that as a result of First Place, individuals will live healthier, happier and more abundant lives with God as their first priority.

A CHRIST-CENTERED HEALTH PROGRAM

Balance

Jesus said, "I have come that they may have life, and have it to the full" (John 10:10). Life becomes abundant when Christ has first place. Abundant living means being in good condition spiritually, mentally, emotionally and physically. That's what First Place is all about. It is a total Christ-centered health program, emphasizing balance in all four areas of life.

Bread

In John 6:35, Jesus described Himself as "the bread of life. He who comes to me will never go hungry." It is through our daily dependence on Jesus that we can achieve balance in all four areas of life. The First Place program is meant to be a daily process. Some days will be better than others, but no matter what, we need to keep Christ in each day and remember that He is the One who satisfies our hunger. How does He do that?

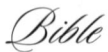

Bible

In Matthew 4:4, Jesus explained that God's Word is central to true satisfaction: "It is written: 'Man does not live on bread alone, but on every word that comes from the mouth of God.'"

One of the main ways God communicates with us is through His Word, the Bible. Studying God's Word reveals guidelines for developing physical well-being, equipping us mentally to make right choices, providing emotional stability to handle everyday circumstances as well as crisis situations, and growing spiritually as we deepen our relationships with Him.

THE NINE COMMITMENTS

The First Place program has Nine Commitments that will help you draw closer to the Lord and aid you in establishing a solid, consistent and healthy Christian life.

To help you achieve growth in all four areas, First Place asks you to keep these Nine Commitments:

1. Attendance
2. Encouragement
3. Prayer
4. Bible reading
5. Scripture memory verse
6. Bible study
7. Live-It plan
8. Commitment Record (CR)
9. Exercise

COMMITMENT ONE: *Attendance*

ATTEND YOUR WEEKLY MEETING

Jesus commanded us in John 13:34 to "Love one another. As I have loved you, so you must love one another." In First Place, you can model love for others by attending a weekly group meeting. Attendance will provide accountability as you seek to reach your First Place goals.

COMMITMENT TWO: *Encouragement*

ENCOURAGE ONE PERSON IN YOUR GROUP WEEKLY

Ecclesiastes 4:12 states: "Though one may be overpowered, two can defend themselves." You are asked to encourage a fellow group member through a phone call, e-mail, fax, postcard, etc. You may also reach out to another group member when you need encouragement.

COMMITMENT THREE: *Prayer*

SET A DAILY TIME FOR PRAYER

God instructs us in Psalm 46:10 to "be still, and know that I am God." You will find a feast of spiritual blessings as you learn to communicate with Him.

- **Group meeting prayer time**—You will spend time in prayer at your weekly meeting. Your prayer requests should be short and specific, relating to your personal needs. All group prayer requests must be kept confidential.

- **Personal prayer time**—Pray daily for fellow members and your leader. Pray also for your own commitments and for God's help in every area of your life.

- **Pray continually**—You can pray at any and all times during the day. Pray when you are tempted in any area of your life. Arm yourself with prayer and watch how God works.

COMMITMENT FOUR: *Bible Reading*

WRITE GOD'S WORD ON YOUR HEART
In Psalm 32:8, God promises, "I will instruct you and teach you in the way you should go; I will counsel you and watch over you." The *First Place Member's Guide* contains a suggested Scripture reading plan that includes a daily selection from both the Old Testament and the New Testament.

In John 8:32, Jesus said, "You will know the truth, and the truth will set you free." The purpose of the Scripture reading commitment is not to study the Bible but to keep you in God's Word daily. Ask God to speak to your heart and allow the Holy Spirit to reveal truths as you make yourself available.

COMMITMENT FIVE: *Scripture Memory Verse*

MEMORIZE ONE VERSE EACH WEEK
Psalm 119:105 states that the Word of God is "a lamp to my feet and a light for my path." God's written Word will be a light to guide your life, but you must know His Word for it to be a light for your path.

As part of the First Place program, you are asked to memorize one verse every week and review it daily. You will quote this verse when you weigh in each week. The memory verse corresponds with the Bible study. Commit it to memory so that you can say along with the psalmist, "I have hidden your word in my heart that I might not sin against you" (Psalm 119:11).

COMMITMENT SIX: *Bible Study*

STUDY GOD'S WORD
Each day you should read, meditate and answer only one day's portion of that week's Bible study. Each week includes five days of Bible study with two days of reflection and review. You will want to come to each group meeting prepared to discuss what truths God has revealed to you that week in Bible study.

COMMITMENT SEVEN: *Live-It Plan*

FOLLOW THE HEALTHY FOOD PLAN CALLED LIVE-IT PLAN
The Live-It plan is a healthy eating plan recommended by credible health professionals. It is designed to help members reach and maintain their healthy weight, meet nutritional requirements, promote good health, lead active lives and reduce chronic disease risks.

The food lists are based on the USDA Food Guide Pyramid. First Place recommends eating three balanced meals each day with optional healthy snacks. In this plan, a well-balanced meal includes certain amounts of foods from each of the following food groups: meats, vegetables, fruits, breads, milk and fats.

AVOID SUGAR AND FOODS WITH ADDED SUGAR
First Place cautions against eating sugar in large amounts and against frequent snacks of foods and beverages containing sugar. Sugary foods supply unnecessary calories and few nutrients.

USING SUGAR SUBSTITUTES
Because of the unknown effects of artificial sweeteners, First Place recommends that members use sugar substitutes in moderation.

COMMITMENT EIGHT:
Commitment Record (cr)

KEEP A RECORD OF YOUR NINE COMMITMENTS
The Commitment Record (CR) is a personal record of the Nine Commitments you keep each week. It is a self-evaluation record that reflects strengths and areas that need improvement. The CR is an accountability tool, not a binding chain. Keeping a record is an opportunity to reflect on how well you are caring for God's temple.

For further reference, you will find a sample CR and instructions on page 16.

COMMITMENT NINE: *Exercise*

EXERCISE THREE TO FIVE TIMES WEEKLY

In 1 Corinthians 3:16, Paul reminded us, "Don't you know that you yourselves are God's temple and that God's Spirit lives in you?" Exercise is maintenance for your body, God's home. For those who need to get fit, the commitment in First Place is to exercise five times each week. For those desiring to maintain fitness, the commitment is a minimum of three times each week. Further, it is recommended that you don't go more than 48 hours without exercising.

The three necessary components of healthy exercise are aerobic activity, strength training and flexibility. The First Place materials will help you evaluate your fitness level and develop a personal exercise plan.

TOOLS *to help you* SUCCEED

Whether you are part of a First Place group or desire to complete the materials alone, the First Place program can help you lose weight and keep it off by helping you develop a healthy lifestyle. The food exchanges, Commitment Records (CRs), Personal Weight Records (PWRs), *First Place Member's Guide* and First Place Bible studies are just a few tools to aid you in your search for wellness. More information about these and other tools is available in the *First Place Member's Guide* or at www.firstplace.org.

FOOD EXCHANGES

Using food exchanges is a simple way to ensure proper nutrition. You can use exchanges for losing weight, gaining weight or maintaining a healthy weight. People can also use food exchanges to regain health lost by years of poor nutrition.

The term "food exchange" doesn't need to be intimidating. Foods are divided into seven exchange lists: bread/starch, meat, vegetable, fruit, milk, fat and free foods.

All the foods within a food list contain approximately the same number of nutrients and calories per serving, which means that one serving of a food from the bread list may be exchanged (or substituted) for one serving of any other item in the bread list.

For example, each of the following would be one bread exchange:

- 1 tortilla
- 1 ½ cups of puffed cereal
- ⅓ cup of peas

By using food exchanges in your daily eating plan, you are always able to choose foods you like that fit your lifestyle. Food exchanges:

- Encourage variety
- Insure well-balanced meals
- Make menu planning easier
- Help establish a permanent lifestyle change

Words of wisdom for those who have joined First Place to lose weight:

- There is no magic potion for losing weight.
- No gimmicks or gadgets can guarantee quick and easy weight loss.
- An effective weight-loss plan needs to be both sensible and livable.

To get long-lasting results, you will need to do the following:

- Eat less, exercise more!
- Change behavior.
- Use portion control.
- Make sure your new habits become a permanent part of your lifestyle.

COMMITMENT RECORDS

Commitment Records will help you keep track of your accomplishments. Each Bible study contains 13 CRs, and they can also be purchased in individually wrapped packages of 13 records each. The following sample will help you complete the blank CR that follows.

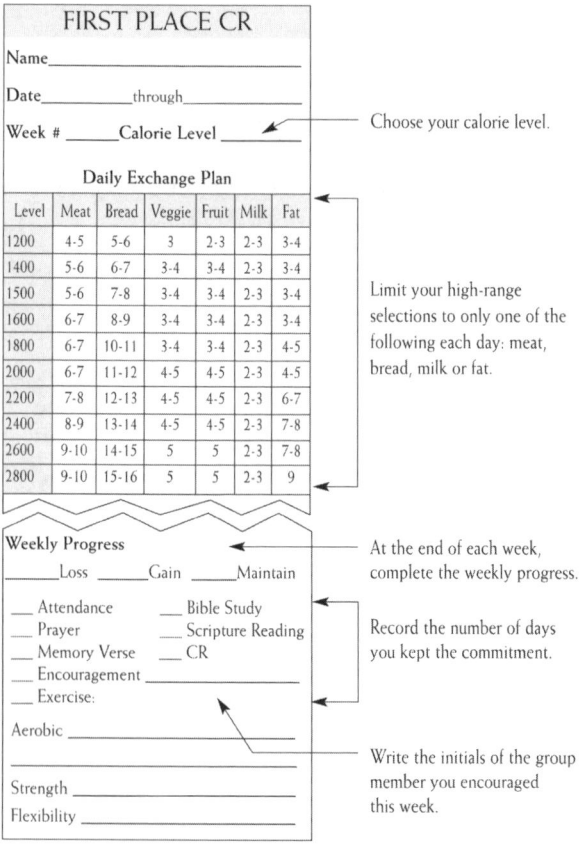

FIRST PLACE CR

Name_____

Date_____through_____

Week # _____Calorie Level _____ — Choose your calorie level.

Daily Exchange Plan

Level	Meat	Bread	Veggie	Fruit	Milk	Fat
1200	4-5	5-6	3	2-3	2-3	3-4
1400	5-6	6-7	3-4	3-4	2-3	3-4
1500	5-6	7-8	3-4	3-4	2-3	3-4
1600	6-7	8-9	3-4	3-4	2-3	3-4
1800	6-7	10-11	3-4	3-4	2-3	4-5
2000	6-7	11-12	4-5	4-5	2-3	4-5
2200	7-8	12-13	4-5	4-5	2-3	6-7
2400	8-9	13-14	4-5	4-5	2-3	7-8
2600	9-10	14-15	5	5	2-3	7-8
2800	9-10	15-16	5	5	2-3	9

Limit your high-range selections to only one of the following each day: meat, bread, milk or fat.

Weekly Progress — At the end of each week, complete the weekly progress.

_____Loss _____Gain _____Maintain

___ Attendance   ___ Bible Study
___ Prayer   ___ Scripture Reading
___ Memory Verse   ___ CR
___ Encouragement _____
___ Exercise:

Aerobic _____

_____

Strength _____

Flexibility _____

Record the number of days you kept the commitment.

Write the initials of the group member you encouraged this week.

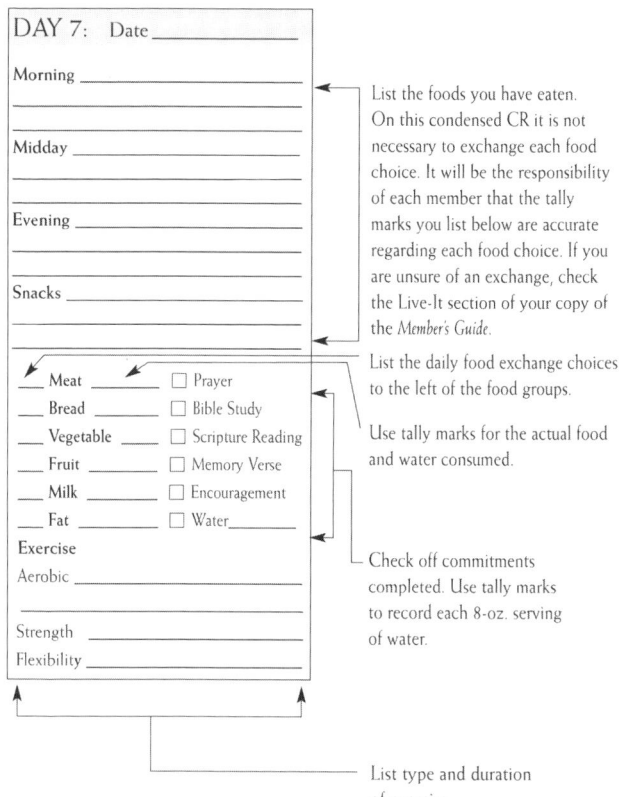

DAY 7: Date _____

Morning _____
_____
_____

Midday _____
_____
_____

Evening _____
_____
_____

Snacks _____
_____
_____

___ Meat _____   ☐ Prayer
___ Bread _____   ☐ Bible Study
___ Vegetable _____   ☐ Scripture Reading
___ Fruit _____   ☐ Memory Verse
___ Milk _____   ☐ Encouragement
___ Fat _____   ☐ Water_____

Exercise
Aerobic _____
_____
Strength _____
Flexibility _____

List the foods you have eaten.
On this condensed CR it is not
necessary to exchange each food
choice. It will be the responsibility
of each member that the tally
marks you list below are accurate
regarding each food choice. If you
are unsure of an exchange, check
the Live-It section of your copy of
the *Member's Guide.*

List the daily food exchange choices
to the left of the food groups.

Use tally marks for the actual food
and water consumed.

Check off commitments
completed. Use tally marks
to record each 8-oz. serving
of water.

List type and duration
of exercise.

PERSONAL WEIGHT RECORDS

Personal Weight Records are another tool to help keep
you on track. By recording your progress each week, the
PWR serves as an ongoing reminder that all your hard
work is paying off. Each Bible Study contains a PWR like
the one on the next page to fill out during the 13 weeks
of that study.

PERSONAL WEIGHT RECORD

Week	Weight	+ or -	Goal This Session	Pounds to Goal
1				
2				
3				
4				
5				
6				
7				
8				
9				
10				
11				
12				
13				
Final				

Beginning Measurements

Waist_____ Hips_____ Thighs_____ Chest_____

Ending Measurements

Waist_____ Hips_____ Thighs_____ Chest_____

THE FIRST PLACE MEMBER'S GUIDE

The *First Place Member's Guide* contains a wealth of information about healthy living and the First Place program, including tips for prayer, journaling and Bible reading; a synopsis of the Live-It plan; an abundance of fitness and activity ideas; a health assessment; information on eating habits, weight gain and obesity; tools for better nutrition and tips to help you maintain your healthy weight. The *First Place Member's Guide* is included in the *First Place Member's Kit*.

FIRST PLACE BIBLE STUDIES

The First Place Bible studies do more than help you fulfill your Nine Commitments. Each study also will teach you about living a healthy lifestyle while helping you grow in your relationship with God. *First Taste* contains samples of several components of a First Place Bible study: teaching, Wellness Worksheets, a Leader's Discussion Guide and menu plans.

TEACHING

The 10-week teaching portion of each Bible study is broken into daily segments that should take about 15 to 20 minutes to complete. The ultimate goal of Bible study is not only for knowledge but also for application and a changed life. You will discuss with your fellow First Place members what you learn each week through this vital exercise. You will find a sample week of teaching beginning on page 21.

WELLNESS WORKSHEETS

The Wellness Worksheets contained in each Bible study are interactive and may be completed on your own or with your group. These worksheets contain helpful information in the spiritual, emotional, physical and mental areas. You will find a sample Wellness Worksheet on page 37.

LEADER'S DISCUSSION GUIDE

A Leader's Discussion Guide is included in the back of each Bible study. This guide helps the group leader build the lessons for the group meetings. A sample week of a Leader's Discussion Guide (corresponding with the sample week of teaching) is on page 60.

MENU PLANS

Each Bible study also includes two weeks of menu plans that incorporate the Live-It plan principles. Many studies also include bonus recipes. You will find a sample week of menu plans beginning on page 42.

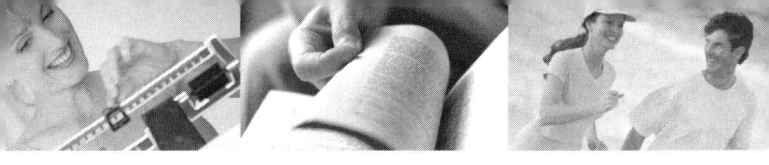

BIBLE STUDY

sample taken from

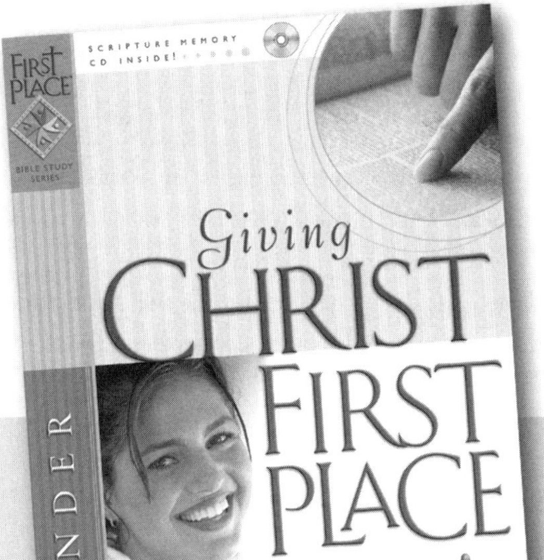

GIVING CHRIST FIRST PLACE

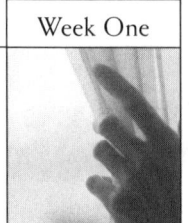

MEMORY VERSE
But seek first his kingdom and his righteousness,
and all these things will be given to you as well.
Matthew 6:33

When embarking upon a journey toward better health,
we need to seek God's help and claim His promises.
In Matthew 22:37 we discover the place God wants to
hold in our lives—*first place*. What a challenge! Loving
God halfheartedly is not enough. He wants complete
commitment, and through that commitment to Him
your life will be forever changed.

In this week's study, you'll have the opportunity to
search your heart and examine your life. Are there areas
of your life you have failed to surrender to Christ? If
Christ is not first place in your thoughts, plans and
actions, what is?

DAY 1: *Time for What You Seek First*

Matthew 6:33 puts the pattern for Christian living in a
nutshell: Seek first the kingdom of God. In your busy
life you cannot do everything. However, the thing you
can decide is what to do first. What you choose first,
over time, takes first place in your life.

If you look at the entries in your calendar or check-book for the past month, you might be surprised by what has been first place in your life lately.

➼ List areas to which you find yourself giving the most time and effort.

God knows that things other than spiritual priorities tend to become the focus of our lives. Your checkbook and calendar will remind you of this fact.

➼ In Matthew 6:25 Jesus mentioned some of the things that divert our attention from His priorities in our lives. What are those things?

Jesus wasn't saying that what you eat, drink or wear is not important; He simply stressed that you need not worry about them. These concerns must never take first place in your life. Instead, Jesus has challenged you to learn some simple lessons about God's provision.

➼ According to Matthew 6:26-30, what does God want you to learn from the birds and flowers?

When you see the lessons of His provision for the birds and flowers, you will begin to understand how

God knows and meets your needs. Philippians 4:19 also reminds you of His promise. He didn't say He would meet some or a few of your needs, but *all* your needs.

➣ Do you believe this promise applies to you? ☐

    ☐ Yes   ☐ No

➣ What needs do you have in your life now that you can turn over to God?

As Christians, the desire to give Christ first place in every area of our lives must be foremost. *Saying* Christ is first and *living* with Christ in first place are different matters. When Christ comes first, your life will change. You will make decisions based on new commitments. You will schedule time based on new priorities.

Use this week's memory verse to keep this commitment in focus. Listen to the CD while exercising. Display the verse in the bathroom and/or kitchen and read it each time you are in that room. Memorizing Scripture will reinforce your commitment to keep Christ in first place and direct your thoughts and actions toward Christ and His kingdom.

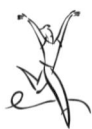
Thank You Lord, for the promise to meet my needs through Your Son, Jesus.

    Lord, help me to trust You and give You first place in my life this week.

DAY 2: *God's Promise . . . Your Choice*

Consider Matthew 6:25-27. When Jesus spoke about "these things" in Matthew 6:33, He was referring to what He said in the verses that preceded verse 33, beginning at verse 25. He offered a choice: 1) worry about these things *or* 2) seek His kingdom. God has promised that we will receive what we need. In spite of this, most Christians continue to worry rather than simply claim this promise. Worry is an affront to God. He told us He would supply all our needs, and He knows what we need even before we ask.

In Matthew 6:28-30, Jesus continued to teach about not worrying about the things of life. Worry is different from being concerned. God wants you to be concerned about others, situations, what is happening in your life and your relationships with others. Pray earnestly about those things, but don't worry and fret over them. If the situation is one over which you have no control, give it to God—He does have control.

⟫ How much time and energy do you give each week to worrying about the things God has promised to provide for those who seek His kingdom first?

When Jesus taught His disciples how to pray in Matthew 6:9-13, part of the prayer focused on the kingdom of God: "Your kingdom come, your will be done on earth as it is in heaven." You will glimpse God's kingdom when His will is done on Earth as it is in heaven.

In Matthew 21:22 we find another wonderful promise from God. When you pray about the things that cause you to worry and when you believe in God's faithfulness, He will provide what you need. What changes would come in your life this day if you asked God to use you to accomplish His will this day in your part of the world—at school, the office, the store or your own home? Allow His kingdom to break through on Earth today through you.

Remember the Serenity Prayer:

God, grant me the serenity to accept the things I cannot change
Courage to change the things I can
And the wisdom to know the difference.
—Reinhold Neibuhr, 1926

As you pray today, list in your prayer journal the details of your worries or concerns and turn them over to Him. Repeat the memory verse in your prayer, telling God that you are willing to seek His kingdom first. Ask Him to help you trust Him more.

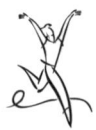

Lord, help me to trust You and to seek You and Your kingdom first.

Lord, help me to focus my energy on things that will make a difference for Your kingdom.

DAY 3: *The Priorities of the Kingdom of God*

Romans 14:17 tells us three things that *are* and two things that *are not* priorities in the kingdom of God.

➤ List the three things that *are* priorities in the kingdom of God.

1.

2.

3.

➤ List the two things that *are not* priorities.

1.

2.

Did you notice that two of these items focus on our physical lives and three of them focus on our spiritual lives? The Bible does not teach that your physical life is unimportant or that it is unnecessary to provide for yourself and those who depend on you.

➤ What do 2 Thessalonians 3:10 and 1 Timothy 5:8 tell us about taking care of responsibilities and physical needs?

While you need to focus on spiritual priorities, you also need to care for your own physical needs and the needs of others. The challenge comes as you attempt to live responsibly without allowing daily pressures to consume all your time and energy. It is our experience that when you nurture your spiritual life, you will find the added emotional energy you need to live in this demanding physical world.

First Corinthians 10:31 gives us a guideline for transforming the activities of everyday life into a lifestyle focused on God and spiritual priorities. Whatever you do during the day, whether eating, drinking or playing, do it all for God's glory.

❧ Write a statement that expresses what "for the glory of God" means to you.

❧ To what degree are you experiencing God's righteousness, joy and peace?

Do you lack the energy needed to be all you can be through the First Place commitments? Use the following prayers to ask for God's help.

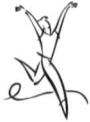

Lord, help me to balance my time and energy to meet the demands of my life today.

Lord, help me to glorify You in all that I do and say this day.

DAY 4: *Commitments to Giving God First Place*

Luke 9:23 contains three commitments we must make if we want to follow Christ with the kingdom of God as our top priority.

≫ What are the commitments Jesus asked His disciples to make?

　1.

　2.

　3.

≫ Describe one area in which you need to deny yourself so you can follow Christ more fully.

≫ What excuses do people use when asked to do something for their church such as teach a class, volunteer in the nursery, visit the sick, answer the telephone, work in the library or any of the many other tasks related to carrying out God's business?

When Jesus told us to take up our cross and follow Him, He meant we were to follow Him wherever He would go. He healed the sick, ministered to those in need, taught His disciples, prayed for sinners, and He depended on His Father to supply all His needs.

If you want to follow Jesus and be like Him, you must be willing to commit yourself to doing the tasks of furthering His kingdom. Seek Him first, and He will help you do all things through Him. Remember Philippians 4:13. Your source of strength is Christ.

Review this week's memory verse.

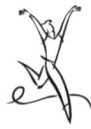

Lord, help me, today, to put my past behind me, take up my cross and follow You.

Lord, show me how to please You in everything I do, including in what I eat and drink.

DAY 5: *Your Spiritual Connection and Evidence*

Matthew 5:16 describes a time when Jesus told His disciples to let their lights shine so that others could see their works and praise their Father in heaven.

➳ Fill in the blanks in the following paragraph:

Jesus assumed that His disciples would live lives that attracted attention. Others would see the_____they did and pay attention to their lives. But Jesus wanted His disciples to do more than attract attention. He wanted people to see their good deeds and_____.

In most cases, people will not make the connection between your good deeds and your Father in heaven unless you help them. You will have to tell them that the reason you live as you do is because of the difference Christ has made in your life. Only then will they glorify God because of your deeds.

>> How would you respond if a coworker or friend said, "You are such a disciplined person! I don't know how you have so much self-control!"?

>> The following verses describe some of the priorities and commitments that indicate you have given Christ first place. Look up each verse and match the verse with the key phrase.

Scripture	Characteristic in Our Lives
a. 1 Samuel 15:22	_____ 1. A desire and willingness to obey God
b. Proverbs 3:9-10	_____ 2. Offering yourself to God as a living sacrifice
c. Romans 12:1	_____ 3. Giving to God from material possessions
d. Romans 13:8	_____ 4. Loving others on an ongoing basis
e. 1 Thessalonians 5:17	_____ 5. An ongoing lifestyle of prayer

✎ Based on these verses, how would you evaluate the degree to which Christ is first place in your life right now? Check the box beside each characteristic that best expresses the degree to which it has developed in your life:

Characteristic in My Life	Strong	Average	Weak
I desire to know and obey God.	☐	☐	☐
I offer myself to God as a living sacrifice.	☐	☐	☐
I give to God from my material possessions.	☐	☐	☐
I love others on an ongoing basis.	☐	☐	☐
I sustain a lifestyle of prayer.	☐	☐	☐
☐ ☐	☐		

In your prayer journal write a prayer for another person in your First Place group and ask God to help this person with whatever needs or struggles he or she is facing. Then write a prayer for a non-Christian who is in your life—such as a neighbor, coworker or family member—and ask the Lord to let the light of God's love in your life shine to others.

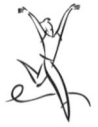

Lord, give me the opportunity to help a friend, family member or coworker make a spiritual connection through my life.

God, give me the wisdom to explain the connection between the way I live and the fact that Jesus is first place in my life.

DAY 6: *Reflections*

You've been studying the Bible for five days; this may be a new experience for you or it may already be a daily part of your life. In either case these studies will help you establish new patterns for your life. Bible study requires a greater priority on the spiritual level of your life than the physical elements of other commitments.

The Reflection section at the end of each week will introduce a powerful spiritual resource—praying through the Scriptures. Whether this is your first or fifth Bible study for First Place, this section will help you overcome those things in your life that have become strongholds. If you are not familiar with praying through Scripture, this section will teach you how. For repeaters, this section will be a refresher and will reiterate those things you've learned.

Praying through Scripture is the process of taking a verse and praying it back to God in your own words. Beth Moore's book *Praying God's Word* explains the process.[1]

You can learn much about letting God be in control and overcoming your own strongholds through Beth Moore's own testimony.

> *I've been educated in the power of God and His Word through field trips of my own failure, weakness, and past bondage. . . I didn't discover what a vital part of my liberation this approach has been until long after I had begun practicing it. I suddenly realized it was no accident that I was finally set free from some areas of*

bondage that had long hindered the abundant, effective, Spirit-filled life in me.[2]

Beth tells us that a stronghold may be an addiction, an unforgiving spirit toward a person who has hurt you, or despair over loss; and it demands so much of your emotional and mental energy that your abundant life is strangled. You, too, can break down the spiritual strongholds in your life as you pray through the Scriptures.[3]

The process isn't complicated: You take a particular verse and pray that verse to the Lord, personalizing the words. The following are examples of praying Scripture. Ask the Lord to reveal the strongholds in your life as you pray each one.

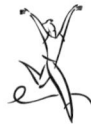

Lord, help me overcome the strongholds in my life. I long for You to be first. I want to seek first Your kingdom and Your righteousness. Thank You for your promise to give me the other things I need (see Matthew 6:33).

Father, when Your words come to me, help me to eat them; make them my joy and my heart's delight, for I bear Your name, O Lord God Almighty (see Jeremiah 15:16).

God, through the victories You give, may Christ's glory be great (see Psalm 21:5).

Day 7: *Reflections*

The key to overcoming strongholds can be found in 2 Corinthians 10:3-5. Consider carefully the meaning of the words. You can pray this Scripture by saying,

> *Lord, You've said I live in the world, but I do not wage*
> *war as the world does. My weapons are not the weapons*
> *of the world. On the contrary, they have divine power*
> *to demolish strongholds. I can demolish arguments and*
> *every pretension that sets itself up against the knowledge*
> *of God; and I take captive every thought to make it*
> *obedient to Christ. Thank You in advance for working*
> *in my life. Amen.*

Before you can tackle the spiritual strongholds in your life, you need to identify the battlefield. As a believer in Jesus, the enemy is waging a constant, personal battle against you, and the primary battlefield is your mind.

Your mind is the control center of your being. Satan tries to make you believe that he is powerful and that you are powerless, and he will try to put destructive and discouraging thoughts in your mind. But you are not powerless; you have God's Holy Spirit living in you. Repeat these words: Nothing is bigger or more powerful than God! The strongest addiction or your worst habit can be overcome through the power of the living God.

The primary goal of your spiritual warfare is found in the verses you just prayed: You need to demolish every argument and pretension that sets itself up against the knowledge of God. You must take your thoughts captive and be obedient to Christ.

As you complete this first week of Bible study, repeat the memory verse. Keep your Scripture memory cards close at hand to help you review. Try saying the verse aloud to a family member or use it in conversation. Each time you use the verse, God will plant this verse more firmly in your mind and heart.

The journey to seek God first begins with a single step. The completion of this first week is a step of progress on that journey. Rejoice at the opportunity to give Christ first place.

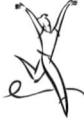

Father God, please help me to keep in mind that my struggle is not against flesh and blood, but against the rulers, against the powers of this dark world and against the spiritual forces of evil in the heavenly realms (see Ephesians 6:12).

Lord, I know I have nothing to fear from my strongholds because You have given me a spirit of power and of love and of a sound mind (see 2 Timothy 1:7).

Lord, thank You for Your protection. Help me to be sober and vigilant because the devil walks around like a lion, seeking whom he may devour. Help me be steadfast in the faith (see 1 Peter 5:8).

Heavenly Father, help me to seek first Your kingdom and Your righteousness, for then all these other things will be given to me (see Matthew 6:33).

Notes
1. Beth Moore, *Praying God's Word* (Nashville, TN: Broadman and Holman, 2000).
2. Ibid., p. 2.
3. Ibid., p. 3.

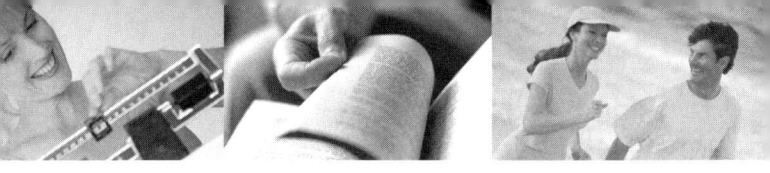

WELLNESS WORKSHEET

sample taken from

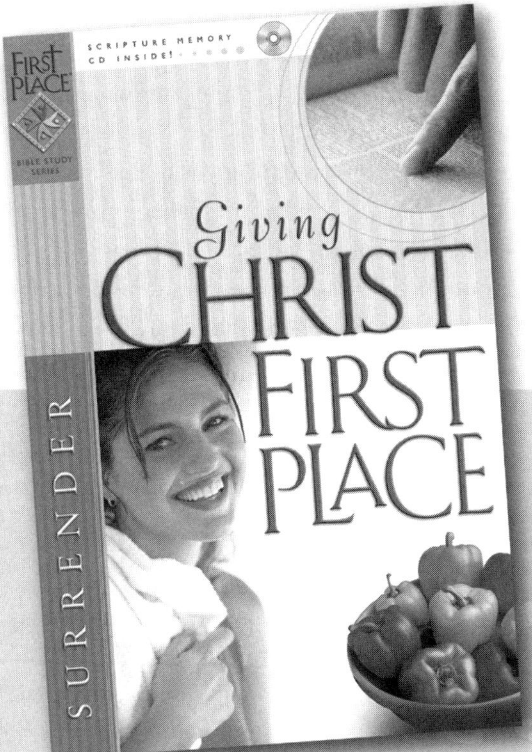

THE AMAZING 10-MINUTE WORKOUT

No time, no fun and *bo-or-or-ring!* These are common reasons people give for not making physical activity a lifetime habit. Yet experts are making it harder and harder to come up with good excuses. The latest recommendations tell us that exercise doesn't have to be hard to be beneficial. In fact, exercise doesn't even have to be exercise! Gone are the days when you had to exercise for at least 30 minutes at a certain heart rate to get the health and fitness benefits of aerobic exercise. What's the exercise prescription for today? "Something is better than nothing, and more is better than something."

The latest recommendations from groups such as the American Heart Association and the American College of Sports Medicine call for at least 30 minutes of moderate physical activity on as many days of the week as possible—preferably every day. The latest twist on this new recommendation is that the activity doesn't have to be done all at one time. Shorter amounts accumulated over the course of a day appear to offer the same health benefits as the more traditional 30 continuous minutes of exercise.

THE BENEFITS OF SHORTER WORKOUTS

Shorter workouts are easier to start and to stick with. It's easy to get burned out on exercise by doing too much too soon. Start slowly and work your way up to longer sessions as your physical activity becomes a habit.

You may also be a person who just doesn't have 30 to 60 minutes to give at one time. Shorter workouts are easier to fit into your schedule and fight boredom by allowing more variety in your routine. They're also great for regular exercisers who occasionally miss or are unable to do their usual routine. When you miss or know you are going to miss a session, just slip in one or two of these shorter workouts wherever and whenever you can.

Are lack of time, lack of enjoyment and boredom among the reasons you have a hard time making exercise a part of your life? Whether you're a regular exerciser or just getting started, think about it. Consider some of the following ideas for fitting 10-minute workouts into your day:

- Walking can be done anywhere, anytime. Think about times in your typical day when you can fit in a short, brisk walk.
- Get up 10 minutes earlier and fit in a quick walk before starting your day.
- Walk as part of your daily quiet time.
- Take 10-minute walking breaks at work.
- Arrive at work 10 minutes early and walk or climb the stairs.
- Take a 10-minute walk around the mall before stopping to shop.
- Walk your dog for 10 minutes.
- Take the entire family out for a 10-minute walk before or after meals.
- Walk around the house during commercials or between shows—you'll easily get in 10 minutes.

Walking is not your only choice. Here are some other creative ideas:

- Pick up the pace when you're doing household chores: 10 minutes of vacuuming, washing the car or working in the yard add up over the course of a day. To get the benefit, however, you have to push the pace a bit. Turn on your favorite music to help keep you moving.
- Buy an exercise videotape and pop it in for 10 minutes.
- Do you have exercise equipment that's collecting dust? Pull it out and try a 10-minute routine instead of feeling like you have to stay on for 30 minutes or longer.
- Rather than just watching your kids play, spend 10 minutes playing with them: shoot baskets, throw a ball or Frisbee, kick a soccer ball, etc.
- Take 10-minute breaks at work and do calisthenics, strength training or stretching exercises.

- Choose a few activities that you enjoy and can do for approximately 10 minutes at a time. Be creative— don't limit yourself to the traditional exercises. Whatever you choose to do, try to make it fun. Remember, the *e* in *exercise* is for *enjoyment!*

✎ Now that you've chosen a few activities, think of some times you can fit them into your day. Think about times in your day when you can be more active, such as when you watch television, shop, work around the house or take a break.

Morning

Noon

Evening

✎ Who can help you free up 10 minutes of time in your daily schedule?

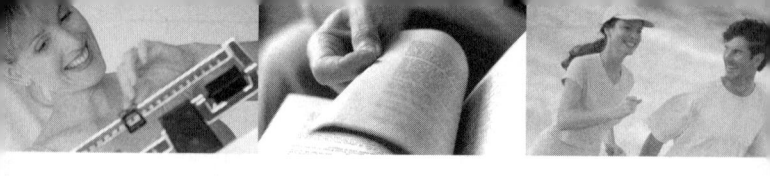

MENU PLANS

sample taken from

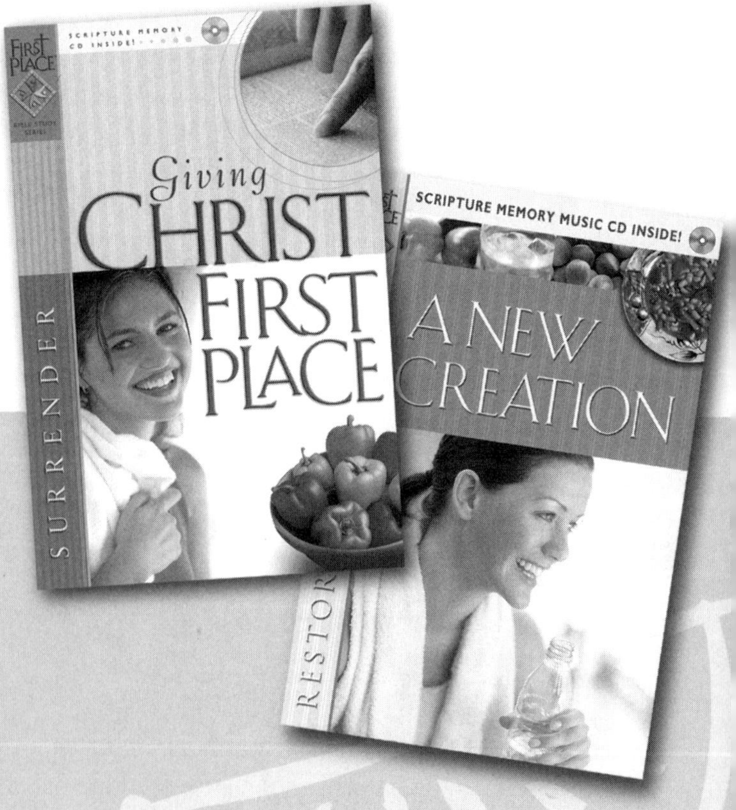

Giving CHRIST FIRST PLACE

SURRENDER

SCRIPTURE MEMORY CD INSIDE!

A NEW CREATION

SCRIPTURE MEMORY MUSIC CD INSIDE!

RESTOR

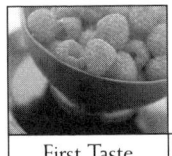

First Taste

FIRST PLACE
MENU PLANS

Each plan is based on approximately 1,400 calories.

Breakfast	0-1 meats, 1-2 breads, 1 fruit, 0-1 milk, 0-½ fat
Lunch	2 meats, 2 breads, 1 vegetable, 1 fruit, 1 fat
Dinner	3 meats, 2 breads, 2 vegetables, 1 fat
Snacks	1 bread, 1 fruit, 1 milk, ½-1 fat (or any remaining exchanges)
Daily Total	4-5 meats, 6-7 breads, 3-4 vegetables, 3-4 fruits, 2-3 milks, 3-4 fats

For more calories, add the following to the 1,400-calorie plan:

1,600 calories	2 breads, 1 fat
1,800 calories	2 meats, 3 breads, 1 vegetable, 1 fat
2,000 calories	2 meats, 4 breads, 1 vegetable, 3 fats
2,200 calories	2 meats, 5 breads, 1 vegetable, 1 fruit, 5 fats
2,400 calories	2 meats, 6 breads, 2 vegetables, 1 fruit, 6 fats

The exchanges for these meals were calculated using the MasterCook software. It uses a database of over 6,000 food items prepared using United States Department of Agriculture (USDA) publications and information from food manufacturers. As with any nutritional program, MasterCook calculates the nutritional values of the recipes based on ingredients. Nutrition may vary due to how the food is prepared, where the food comes from, soil content, season, ripeners, processing and methods of preparation. For these reasons, please use the recipes and menu plans as approximate guides. As always, consult your physician and/or a registered dietitian before starting a diet program.

Menu Plans for Two Weeks

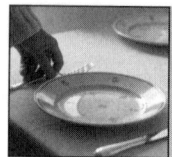

Note: We've included bonus recipes in this study's menu plans. Recipes for *italicized* items in menus can be found in each mealtime section.

🍎 Breakfast

⅓ medium cantaloupe or honeydew melon, topped with

1 c. artificially sweetened pineapple-flavored nonfat yogurt and

¼ c. Grape Nuts cereal

Exchanges: 1 ½ breads, 1 fruit, 1 milk

~ ~

Turkey Bacon, Potato and Egg Scramble

1 small banana

1 6-oz. container artificially sweetened nonfat yogurt (any flavor)

Exchanges: 1 meat, 1 bread, 1 fruit, 1 milk, ½ fat

1   packet Quaker Extra instant oatmeal
1   slice whole-wheat toast
½   medium banana
1   tsp. peanut butter
1   c. nonfat milk
Exchanges: 2 breads, 1 fruit, 1 milk, ½ fat

~ ~

Bonus Breakfast Recipes

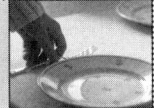

Biscuits with Sausage Gravy

6   oz. bulk turkey sausage
1   7½-oz. can (10 ct.) reduced-fat buttermilk biscuits
2   c. nonfat milk
2   tbsp. all-purpose flour
2   tsp. butter-flavored flakes (such as Molly McButter)
¼   tsp. black pepper
    Nonstick cooking spray

Preheat oven to 450° F. Arrange biscuits on nonstick baking sheet and set aside. Heat skillet coated with cooking spray over medium heat; crumble sausage into skillet and cook until thoroughly done. Drain any visible fat; return to skillet. When sausage is nearly done, combine milk, flour, butter-flavored flakes and pepper in medium bowl; mix well and add to skillet with sausage. Cook 8 minutes or until thickened, stirring occasionally with spatula to prevent sticking.

While gravy is cooking, place biscuits in oven; bake 5 to 6 minutes or until done. Split biscuits and arrange 4 halves on each serving plate; top with $\frac{1}{2}$ cup sausage gravy. Serves 5.

Exchanges: $\frac{1}{2}$ meat, 2 breads, $\frac{1}{2}$ milk, 1 fat

~~~~~~~~~~~~~~~~~~~~~~~~~~~~~~~~~~~~~~

Cranberry-Cinnamon Scones with Fresh Peaches and Vanilla Cream

1	c. plus 6 tbsp. nonfat milk, divided
1	tbsp. cornstarch
3	tbsp. Splenda sugar substitute, divided
1	tbsp. vanilla extract
1	c. plus 2 tbsp. Bisquick reduced-fat baking mix
2	tbsp. dried cranberries
1	tbsp. sugar
$\frac{1}{2}$	tsp. ground cinnamon
$\frac{1}{8}$	tsp. ground nutmeg
2	tbsp. reduced-calorie margarine, melted
2	c. sliced fresh peaches
	Butter-flavored nonstick cooking spray

Whisk together 1 cup milk, cornstarch and 2 tablespoons Splenda in medium saucepan until well blended. Cook over medium-high heat, stirring constantly until thickened. Remove from heat, stir in vanilla and let cool; transfer vanilla cream to refrigerator to chill.

Preheat oven to 450° F. In large mixing bowl, combine baking mix, cranberries, sugar, remaining

Splenda, cinnamon and nutmeg; blend well. Add
remaining milk and margarine; stir until just blended.
Spoon batter onto nonstick baking sheet coated
with cooking spray, creating 4 triangular mounds.
Bake 10 to 12 minutes or until lightly browned.
Remove from oven and serve each topped with ½
cup sliced peaches and ¼ cup chilled vanilla cream.
Serves 4.
Exchanges: 2 breads, ½ fruit, ½ milk, 1 fat

~~~~~~~~~~~~~~~~~~~~~~~~~~~~~~~~~~~~~~

Turkey Bacon, Potato and Egg Scramble

- 2 slices turkey bacon, crisply cooked and crumbled
- ⅓ lb. small red potatoes (about 2 potatoes), cubed
- 2 medium eggs, slightly beaten (or ½ c. egg substitute)
- 1 c. water
- 2 tbsp. nonfat milk
  Dash salt
  Dash pepper
- 2 tsp. reduced-calorie margarine
- 2 tsp. sliced green onions
- 1 tsp. diced pimientos

Bring water and potatoes to boil in small saucepan.
Let cook 6 to 8 minutes or until tender; drain and
set aside. In small bowl, beat together eggs (or egg
substitute), milk, salt and pepper with fork; set aside.
Preheat medium skillet over medium-high heat and
add margarine. Sauté potatoes 3 to 4 minutes until

slightly browned; add green onions and pimientos. Cook 1 minute more, stirring constantly. Pour egg mixture over potato mixture. As the mixture begins to set, gently stir until the uncooked eggs begin to cook and set. Cook 2 to 3 minutes or until eggs are cooked but moist. Sprinkle with crumbled bacon and serve. Serves 2.

Exchanges: 2 breads, ½ fat

🍎 LUNCH

Quick and Crunchy Chicken Salad

8	oz. diced cooked chicken breast
1	16-oz. pkg. shredded cabbage with carrots slaw mix
¼	c. sliced red onion
1	3-oz. pkg. ramen noodles, crumbled
½	c. bottled Wish-Bone Citrus Splash vinaigrette salad dressing
1	15-oz. can mandarin orange sections, drained
4	c. chopped romaine lettuce

Time-Saving Tip: No time to bake a chicken? Many grocery stores offer roasted whole chickens in their deli department. Remember to remove the skin before using the chicken for recipes, and keep unused portion refrigerated.

Combine chicken, slaw mix and red onion in large bowl. Add crumbled ramen (save seasoning packet for another use). Pour dressing over top; toss well to coat. Gently stir in mandarin orange sections. Spoon equal amounts onto each of four 1-cup servings of chopped lettuce. Serves 4.

Serve each with a 1-ounce breadstick.

Exchanges: 2 meats, 1 bread, 2 vegetables, ½ fruit, 1 fat

~~~~~~

Soup and Sandwich

1   c. Healthy Choice garden vegetable soup
    Peanut-butter sandwich, made with
2   slices diet whole-wheat bread and
1   tbsp. peanut butter
1   small banana

Exchanges: 1 meat, 2 breads, 2 vegetables, 1 fruit, 1 fat

~~~~~~

Lean Cuisine Deluxe French Bread Pizza

Serve with 1 serving *Easy Coleslaw.*

Exchanges: 1 ½ meats, 2 ½ breads, 1 vegetable, ½ fruit, 1 fat

~~~~~~

Mediterranean-Style Seafood and Pasta Salad

6   oz. cooked salad shrimp
1 ½ c. miniature pasta shells
1   c. halved grape tomatoes
1   c. diced zucchini
½   c. sliced mushrooms

$\frac{1}{4}$ c. ripe olives (pits removed)

4 oz. Mediterranean-style feta cheese, crumbled

$\frac{1}{2}$ c. low-fat balsamic vinaigrette salad dressing

4 c. fresh spinach leaves

Cook pasta according to package directions, omitting salt and fat. Drain and rinse; place in large bowl. Add shrimp, tomatoes, zucchini, mushrooms, olives and feta cheese; stir to combine. Add salad dressing; toss to coat. Arrange 1 cup spinach leaves on each serving plate; top with shrimp mixture. Serves 4.

Serve each with 1 cup green grapes.

Exchanges: 2 meats, 2 breads, 1 vegetable, 1 fruit, 1 fat

BONUS LUNCH RECIPES

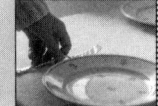

Easy Coleslaw

1 16-oz. pkg. shredded cabbage with carrots

1 c. nonfat mayonnaise

$\frac{1}{4}$ c. apple cider vinegar

1 tbsp. honey

1 tsp. celery seeds

$\frac{1}{4}$ c. raisins

Place cabbage mixture in large bowl; set aside. In small bowl, combine mayonnaise, vinegar and honey; blend well and pour over cabbage. Toss to coat. Add celery seeds and raisins; toss again. Refrigerate until ready to serve. Serves 8.

Exchanges: $\frac{1}{2}$ vegetable, $\frac{1}{2}$ fruit

Orange-Glazed Carrots and Grapes

- 2 10-oz. pkgs. frozen whole baby carrots
- 1 tbsp. brown sugar
- 2 tsp. cornstarch
- 1/4 tsp. ground ginger
- 1/8 tsp. salt
- 3/4 c. unsweetened orange juice
- 1 c. seedless red grapes, halved

Cook carrots according to package directions, omitting salt; set aside. Combine brown sugar, cornstarch, ginger and salt in saucepan. Use wire whisk to gradually stir in orange juice; bring to boil over medium heat. Cook 1 minute, stirring constantly; stir in carrots and grapes. Cook 2 minutes more or until heated through, stirring occasionally. Serves 4.
Exchanges: 2 vegetables, ½ fruit

☕ DINNER

Steak with Mushroom Sauce

- 2 2-in.-thick beef tenderloin steaks (about 1 lb. total), trimmed of fat
  Salt and pepper to taste
- 1 tsp. olive oil
- 8 oz. mushrooms, sliced (can use baby portobello and/or button)
- 1/4 c. beef consommé
- 1/4 c. whipping cream
- 2 tsp. Dijon mustard

Season steaks with salt and pepper on both sides; set aside. Preheat oil in large skillet over medium heat; add steaks and cook to desired doneness, turning once (about 10 minutes total for medium-rare and 14 minutes for medium). Transfer steaks to a warm platter. Use same skillet to cook mushrooms 4 minutes over medium heat. Stir in consommé, cream and mustard. Cook and stir over medium heat 2 to 3 minutes or until slightly thickened. Add more seasoning to taste, if desired. Slice each steak into 6 pieces; place 3 pieces on each of 4 plates. Top each with 2 tablespoons mushroom sauce. Serves 4.

Serve each with 1 *Twice-Baked Broccoli Potato* and a 1-ounce dinner roll.

Exchanges: 3 meats, 2 breads, 1 ½ vegetables, 1 ½ fats

~ ~

Italian Grilled Chicken

   4   boneless, skinless chicken breasts (about 1 lb.)
   ¾   c. low-fat Italian salad dressing

Place chicken breasts and dressing in large sealable plastic bag. Refrigerate 3 hours or overnight. When ready to use, remove breasts from dressing and grill over medium heat 8 minutes; turn and grill 4 to 5 minutes more or until chicken is no longer pink. Serves 4.

Serve each with 1 serving *Grilled Vegetable Kabobs* (including 3 grilled tomatoes) and 1 serving *Garlic Mashed Potatoes.*

Exchanges: 3 meats, 1 bread, 2 vegetables, 1 fat

Fish Fillets Florentine au Gratin

    4   5-oz. tilapia or other firm white-fish fillets
    ¼   tsp. lemon-pepper seasoning
    1   10-oz. pkg. frozen creamed spinach, thawed
    ¼   c. fine dry Italian bread crumbs
    ¼   c. shredded 2% cheddar cheese
        Nonstick cooking spray

Preheat oven to 400° F. Season fillets with lemon-pepper seasoning and arrange on nonstick baking sheet coated with cooking spray; set aside. In small bowl, combine thawed spinach with bread crumbs; spoon mixture evenly over fillets and bake 15 minutes or until fish flakes easily. Top each fillet with 1 tablespoon cheese and bake 1 to 2 minutes more or until cheese is melted. Serves 4.

Serve each with 1 serving *Sweet Potatoes and Sugar Snap Peas*.

Exchanges: 3 meats, 2 breads, 2 vegetables, 1 fat

~~~~~~

Mexican Restaurant Fajitas

    ½   order chicken or steak fajitas
    2   flour tortillas
    ½   c. refried beans
    ½   c. salsa
    1   tsp. sour cream

Exchanges: 3 to 4 meats, 3 breads, 2 vegetables, 2 fats

~~~~~~

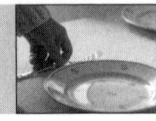

Cocktail Sauce

½   c. no-salt-added tomato sauce
2   tbsp. minced fresh chives
2   tbsp. ketchup
2   tbsp. chili sauce
1   tbsp. fresh lemon juice
2   tsp. prepared horseradish
6   drops Tabasco sauce

In small bowl, combine tomato sauce, chives, ketchup, chili sauce, lemon juice, horseradish and Tabasco. Serves 4.

Exchanges: Free

~ ~

Garlic Mashed Potatoes

3   c. peeled and cubed baking potatoes
1 to 2 tsp. chopped garlic
    Water
¼   c. fat-free half-and-half
1   tbsp. reduced-calorie margarine
¼   tsp. salt
    Dash pepper

Place potatoes and garlic in large saucepan; cover with water and bring to boil. Reduce heat; simmer 20 minutes. Drain and return to pan. Add half-and-half, margarine, salt and pepper to taste. To beat potato mixture, use electric mixer set on medium speed. Serves 4.

Exchanges: 1 bread, ½ fat

~ ~

Twice-Baked Broccoli Potatoes

    2   medium-sized baking potatoes (about ¾ lb.)
    2   c. frozen broccoli florets
    1   tbsp. low-fat sour cream
    1   tbsp. reduced-calorie margarine
        Salt and pepper to taste
    1   tbsp. shredded 2% cheddar cheese

Wash potatoes and prick skin several times with fork. Place in microwave-safe dish and microwave on high 5 minutes; turn potatoes over and cook 4 minutes more. Let sit 2 minutes; slice in half lengthwise. Scoop out pulp (being careful not to tear surrounding skin) into medium bowl. Add broccoli, sour cream, margarine, and salt and pepper to taste. Mix well and refill skins with pulp mixture. Top with cheese and microwave 2 to 3 minutes. Serves 4.

Exchanges: 1 bread, 1 vegetable, ½ fat

☕ SNACKS AND DESSERTS

Apple Cobbler

    6   medium apples, peeled, cored and thinly sliced
    1   6-oz can frozen apple juice concentrate,
        unsweetened and undiluted

2	tbsp. cornstarch
3	tbsp. reduced-fat margarine, divided
1	tsp. cinnamon
1	tsp. vanilla extract
½	c. flour
⅛	tsp. salt
⅛	tsp. nutmeg

Preheat oven to 350° F. In a medium saucepan, combine apple juice and cornstarch; cook over medium heat until thick and bubbly. Sir in 1 tablespoon margarine, cinnamon and vanilla extract; add apples and toss to coat. Pour into 9-inch pie plate; set aside. In a separate bowl, mix together flour, salt, nutmeg and 2 tablespoons margarine until crumbly; sprinkle over apple mixture. Bake 30 minutes. Excellent served warm. Serves 8.

Exchanges: 1 ½ fruits, ½ bread, ½ fat

~ ~

Banana Milk Shake

1	frozen banana (peel before freezing)
1	c. nonfat milk
1	packet artificial sweetener
1	tbsp. fat-free whipped topping

Break frozen banana into pieces and place in blender. Add milk and sweetener; blend until smooth. Serve topped with whipped topping. Serves 1.

Exchanges: 2 fruits, 1 milk

CONVERSION CHART

equivalent IMPERIAL *and* METRIC *measurements*

Liquid Measures

Fluid Ounces	U.S.	Imperial	Milliliters
	1 teaspoon	1 teaspoon	5
$\frac{1}{4}$	2 teaspoons	1 dessert spoon	7
$\frac{1}{2}$	1 tablespoon	1 tablespoon	15
1	2 tablespoons	2 tablespoons	28
2	$\frac{1}{4}$ cup	4 tablespoons	56
4	$\frac{1}{2}$ cup or $\frac{1}{4}$ pint		110
5		$\frac{1}{4}$ pint or 1 gill	140
6	$\frac{3}{4}$ cup		170
8	1 cup or $\frac{1}{2}$ pint		225
9			250 or $\frac{1}{4}$ liter
10	1 $\frac{1}{4}$ cups	$\frac{1}{2}$ pint	280
12	1 $\frac{1}{2}$ cups or $\frac{3}{4}$ pint		340
15		$\frac{3}{4}$ pint	420
16	2 cups or 1 pint		450
18	2 $\frac{1}{4}$ cups		500 or $\frac{1}{2}$ liter
20	2 $\frac{1}{2}$ cups	1 pint	560
24	3 cups or 1 $\frac{1}{2}$ pints		675
25		1 $\frac{1}{4}$	700
30	3 $\frac{3}{4}$ cups	1 $\frac{1}{2}$ pints	840
32	4 cups		900
36	4 $\frac{1}{2}$ cups		1,000 or 1 liter
40	5 cups	2 pints or 1 quart	1,120
48	6 cups or 3 pints		1,350
50		2 $\frac{1}{2}$ pints	1,400

Solid Measures

U.S. and Imperial Measures		Metric Measures	
Ounces	Pounds	Grams	Kilos
1		28	
2		56	
3 ½		100	
4	¼	112	
5		140	
6		168	
8	½	225	
9		250	¼
12	¾	340	
16	1	450	
18		500	½
20	1 ¼	560	
24		675	
27		750	¾
32	2	900	
36	2 ¼	1,000	1
40	2 ½	1,100	
48	3	1,350	
54		1,500	1 ½
64	4	1,800	
72	4 ½	2,000	2
80	5	2,250	2 ¼
100	6	2,800	2 ¾

Oven Temperature Equivalents

Fahrenheit	Celsius	Gas Mark	Description
225	110	$\frac{1}{4}$	Cool
250	130	$\frac{1}{2}$	
275	140	1	Very Slow
300	150	2	
325	170	3	Slow
350	180	4	Moderate
375	190	5	
400	200	6	Moderately Hot
425	220	7	Fairly Hot
450	230	8	Hot
475	240	9	Very Hot
500	250	10	Extremely Hot

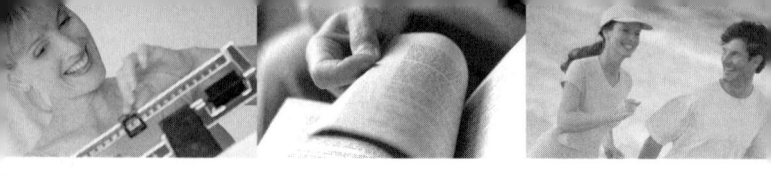

LEADER'S DISCUSSION GUIDE

sample taken from

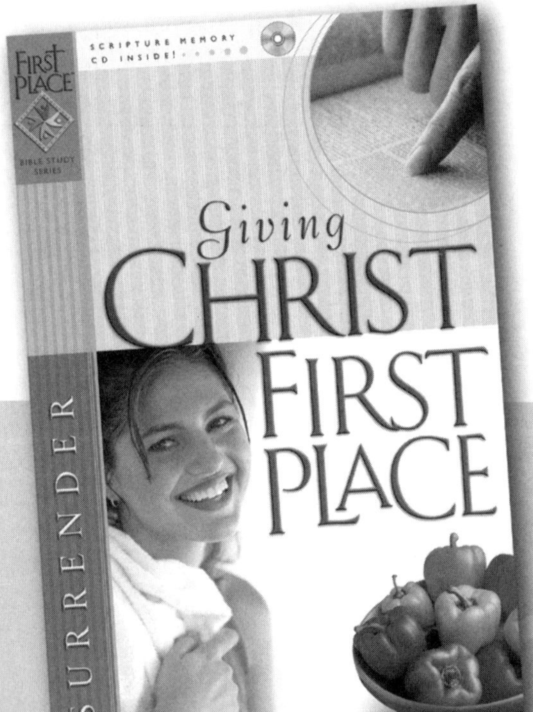

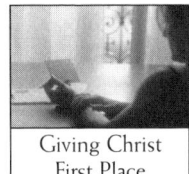

LEADER'S DISCUSSION GUIDE

Giving Christ
First Place

Week One: Giving Christ First Place

1. Ask a volunteer to recite Matthew 6:33 from memory. Form groups of three to share what members discovered about their lives by looking at their checkbooks and calendars for the last month.

2. On the board write the headings "Lessons from the Birds" and "Lessons from the Flowers." Bring the whole group together and have someone read Matthew 6:26-28; then invite members to share what they wrote about these lessons on Day 1. Have a volunteer write key ideas on the board as others share.

3. Read Luke 9:23. Have members return to their groups of three and refer to their material on Day Four, page 15. Ask them to share with their small groups what they wrote about the three commitments in Luke 9:23. Allow 10 to 12 minutes for this discussion.

4. With the whole group back together, have someone read 1 Corinthians 10:31. Explain: Our goal is to do all we do for the glory of God. Discuss how the work they are doing in the First Place program can bring glory to God.

5. In the weeks ahead, as members make progress in reaching their goals, opportunities will come to help them make a spiritual connection. Have someone read Matthew 5:16. Have two volunteers role-play

a situation in which one compliments the other on weight loss. In the first case, the person makes no attempt to make a spiritual connection. In the second, the person tries to help the other see the spiritual connection.

6. Discuss the concept of using Scripture for prayer. Use examples from Day 6 or Day 7. Ask for volunteers to say a sentence prayer from their favorite Bible verse. Write this week's memory verse on the board in the form of a prayer, as on Day Seven.

7. Lead the whole group in a closing time of prayer. Ask them to thank God for the progress He will help them make in reaching their goals. Close the prayer time by asking God to use group members to bring Him glory as they deal with their health-related challenges.

CONTRIBUTORS

Jodi Wilkinson, M.D., M.S., the writer of the Wellness Worksheet for this sampler, is a physician and exercise physiologist at the Cooper Institute in Dallas, Texas. He trained at the University of Texas Health Science Center in San Antonio, Texas, and Baylor University Medical Center in Dallas. Dr. Wilkinson conducts research on physical activity, nutrition and weight management and has worked with the American Heart Association to develop a health program. He believes strongly in using biblical teaching to motivate people to take care of their physical bodies and enjoy abundant living. Jody and his wife, Natalie, have been married nearly 15 years and have two daughters, Jordan and Sarah, and twin sons, Joel and Cooper.

Scott Wilson, C.P.C., C.E.C., A.A.C., the author of the menu plans for this study, is the national food consultant for First Place. Scott is a certified personal chef with the United States Personal Chef Association (USPCA) and is currently serving in the USPCA as chair of the National Advisory Council. He is also a certified executive chef, member of the American Academy of Chefs (AAC) and a member of the American Culinary Federation (ACF). In addition to his role as a personal chef, Scott also serves as an instructor for the Culinary Business Academy of Atlanta, is on the Culinary Advisory Board of the Art Institute of Atlanta and has recently become the Southeast demonstrator chef for AGA Ranges USA. Scott has published three cookbooks and lives in Cumming, Georgia, with his wife, Jennifer, and their daughter, Katie.